kotobuki

the 10 keys of Okinawa

to live happy

"Nifedebiru" (which means "thank you" in the Okinawan language), I sincerely thank

my wife, my children, family and friends, for their encouragement

the Okinawans, for their patience, their sharing and their kindness

the Bushido dojos in Landerneau and Okinawa Karatedō Kobudō Shōrin-ryū Bushinkan, Nanjo, for their support

Nanjo City Hall for insights into Okinawa culture, history and way of life

Hesna Cailliau, author, speaker and expert in Asian culture, for her kindness and for the preface to the book

about the author

a karateka who improvises himself as a writer ...

after a family trip ...

with the wish to share a certain art of living observed on site in Okinawa

In his book, Hervé Stéphanus reconnects with the tradition of travel writers: the joy of a trip is not in the fact of managing to complete the circuit of a tour operator but in the unexpected surprises that arise along the way while taking his time. And it is what the author shares with his readers for their greatest happiness.

By spending several consecutive weeks in Okinawa, a name that evokes for the West a bloody battle in the Pacific, Hervé shows us all the difference between the knowledge that is acquired at the stroke of a plan and the knowledge that arises from heart-to-heart exchanges with people encountered on site. It emerges from this field experience, the discovery of traditions in reverse of ours and still alive: it is because the inhabitants of Okinawa knew how to keep them intact, that they were able to face the hazards and the tragedies of their history and maintain their self-confidence, which has enabled them to bounce back from each disaster: "Seven times on the ground, and each time back on their feet" goes the saying.

This "small" population offers us 10 keys to living happy, very largely inspired by a "mix of ancestral cultures", which are added those of neighboring countries. From Confucianism, they retained the respect for the Ancients and the love of work which rhymes with service: happiness is in the bond more than in the good; from Buddhism the value of the present moment, allowing to enjoy life: "carpe diem"; from their own culture, they inherited karate and its credo "a healthy mind in a healthy body", as well as communion with nature.

The Okinawans implicitly invite us to reconnect with our own traditions, to find the gold nuggets buried under the dust of time because people cut off from its roots loses faith in its future. Traditions and progress, far from being opposed, mutually enrich each other. Being well rooted in its traditions makes you want to go see what is happening elsewhere and be inspired by it, while keeping its uniqueness. Hervé gives us a good example of it here.

Hesna Cailliau

During a family trip, we decided to go to Okinawa. On one hand because it is the cradle of karate (I am a karate practitioner), on the other hand because it is a place at the crossroads of Chinese, Taiwanese, Korean and Japanese cultures.

Once there, we discovered that there was indeed a strong anchoring in karate and multiculturalism, but also an art of living specific to Okinawa, an art of living that exudes happiness.

For tourists visiting Asia, travel agencies often offer only two days of Okinawa sightseeing. For our part, we wanted to spend several consecutive weeks there, to live as much as possible in the company of Okinawans, to immerse ourselves and understand things.

We thus discovered that Okinawa has a particular history, has secrets and a philosophy of life that is undoubtedly unique in the world.

I then wanted to share this experience with this book written mainly on site during our stay (often early in the morning), supplemented by several studies and put into shape after our return.

The Ryū-kyū archipelago is located between Taiwan, China, Korea and Japan, with, thus, multiple influences from these different countries. The culture of Okinawa is also called "chanpurū of cultures", ie a mix of different cultures.

The three kingdoms then forming the kingdom of Ryū-kyū which were regularly at war were unified in 1429 by Sho Hashi. Sho Hashi was originally from the Nanjo region in the southeast of the island.

Sho Hashi did not come from a royal line, but was a "simple" citizen, which is quite unique in itself and even more so at the time.

Another peculiarity, the Ryū-kyū kingdom was organized in a matriarchal way. Women indeed played the leading role, with the high priestesses in particular, called the kimi, who were often members of the royal family. The kimi prayed for the people to be healthy and for crops to be abundant.

The Ryū-kyū kingdom thus enjoyed great prosperity thanks to its political stability and its central geographical location, allowing strong commercial and cultural ties with neighboring countries, particularly China.

For several decades, there was indeed a commercial but also strong cultural proximity between the Ryū-kyū kingdom and the Chinese Ming dynasty.

Under the reign of Sho Shin (1477-1526), king of the Ryū-kyū kingdom, a decree established a confucianist state. Sho Shin wanted a peaceful society. The population was then forbidden to own weapons. Which was quite unusual at this time.

In the spring of 1609, Okinawa was invaded by 3,000 Satsuma samurai, who came from the Japanese island of Kyūshū.

The samurai of Satsuma did not meet much opposition as possession of weapons was not allowed. The samurai took rapidly the advantage, especially at Shuri Castle, palace of kings.

Japanese representatives of the Satsuma tightened the ban on the possession of weapons in Okinawa.

Thus, during these years without authorization to hold a weapon, the inhabitants of Okinawa learned to defend themselves with bare-handed techniques, partly from China, as well as with agrarian tools, the whole undoubtedly constituting the premises of the karate (initially "to-de", "hand of China") and kobudō.

The kingdom of Ryū-kyū, whose center was Shuri Castle, came under the tutorship of the Japanese shogun and then lost much of its independence.

The French navigator La Pérouse was the first to pilot an expedition which passed through the Ryū-kyū Islands with his two ships, L'Astrolabe and La Boussole, on May 4, 1787. The crews were able to have friendly exchanges with the islanders. In his diary, La Pérouse notes that he is "rather inclined to believe" that in "the great island of Likeu" (Ryū-kyū), the Europeans "would be received and would perhaps find a trade there as advantageous as in Japan. ".

During his exile in Saint Helena, around 1815, Napoleon I was informed by the navigator Basil Hall that there was in Okinawa a peaceful kingdom in which weapons were not authorized. Napoleon could not imagine that a people could know neither war, nor weapon. This episode relating to Napoleon is well known to Okinawans.

Okinawa became the 47th prefecture of Japan in 1879. Sho Tai, the last king of the Ryū-kyū kingdom was deposed at that time.

During World War II, the Battle of Okinawa was initially scheduled to last three days. It actually lasted three months, from April 1 to June 22, 1945. This battle opposed the USA (represented by General Buckner, who died during the battle) and Japan (represented by General Ushijima, who put an end to his days just before the end of the battle).

These clashes resulted in around 215,000 deaths (including approximately 150,000 Okinawans, engaged or civilians, approximately 50,000 Japanese soldiers and 15,000 American soldiers).

At the end of the war, and before taking his own life, Japanese Admiral Minoru Ota sent a telegram to the Japanese Military Staff requesting that Japan may have special consideration for the Okinawans, in view of their situation and their courage during the war.

This is considered the bloodiest battle in the Pacific. It seems that the Japanese military has portrayed the US military in such a way that it causes many residents from Okinawa to throw themselves off the cliffs, or even collectively blow themselves up in the caves used as a refuge, rather than becoming prisoners of the Americans.

The extreme violence of the fighting and the bitter struggle of the Japanese defense in Okinawa would have radically called into question the American plan to conquer Japan and would have led the Americans to decide on the use of the atomic bomb in Hiroshima and Nagasaki to bring the Japan to stop the war.

The inhabitants of Okinawa were not, a priori and at the time, really considered by the Japanese.

Then, Okinawa became American after the Second World War, from September 7, 1945. The USCAR (United States Civil Administration of Ryū-kyū Islands) gradually settled.

The USA has set up sporting events, supplying equipment for schools etc. American culture has thus spread around the bases of GIs.

Okinawa became Japanese again on May 15, 1972. This had several consequences, for example the change from dollar to yen, driving on the right to driving on the left etc.

These many changes brought immigration from Okinawa to other countries, such as Brazil and the USA including Hawaii.

Without a king from 1979, Shuri Castle was used as a school and as a sanctuary until 1945. During World War II, the castle was destroyed, before being restored in the 1970s to gradually become a place. touristic.

Thanks to the historical fidelity of its reconstruction, Shuri Castle was classified as a UNESCO World Heritage Site in November 2000, along with the architectural ensemble that surrounds it.

A few months earlier, on July 22, 2000, Shuri Castle hosted the 26th G8 summit. A photo was taken in front of Shuri Palace on this occasion in the presence of Tony Blair, Bill Clinton, Jean Chrétien, Gerhard Schroeder, Yoshiro Mori, Vladimir Poutine, Romano Prodi, Guiliano Amato and Jacques Chirac.

On October 31, 2019, a fire ravaged the castle. In the past, including medieval times, the castle had already been destroyed several times and always rebuilt.

"Nana korobi yaoki" is a proverb which translates in French as "falls seven times, but, each time, get up".

For several decades, the link between many countries and Okinawa has strengthened thanks to the development of karate, which brings many karateka to Okinawa every year, and reciprocally with Okinawans karateka who visit regularly in many countries around the world.

Finally, "Uchina-Guchi", the language of Okinawa, which is different from Japanese, continues to be spoken even today by Okinawans, called in their language "Uchinanchu".

"Thank you", for example, is "arigatô" in Japanese and "nifedebiru" in the Okinawan language.

The same goes for "welcome", which is called "yokoso" in Japanese and "mensore" in the Okinawan language.

Or for "hello" which is said "konnichiwa" in Japanese and "haisai" for men or "haitai" for women, in the language of Okinawa.

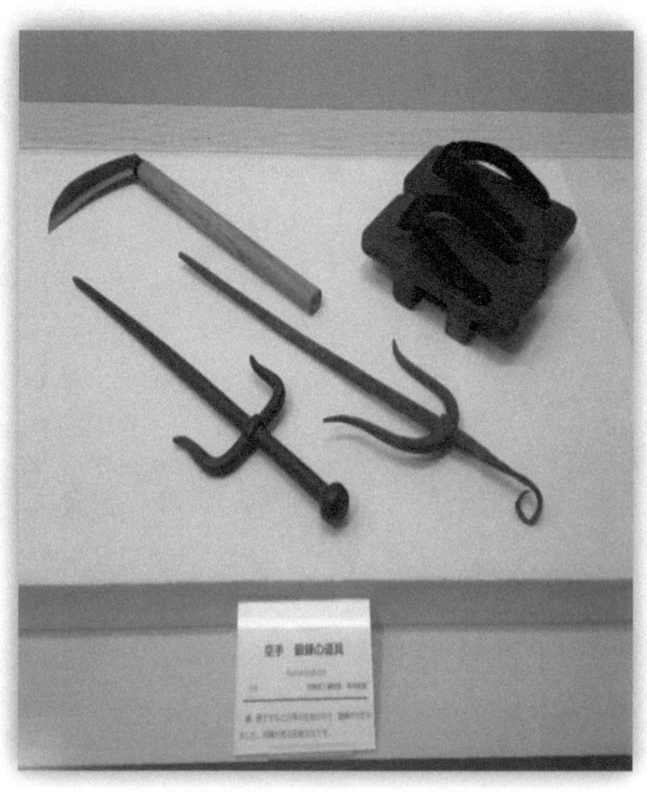

Photos, among others, of Sai, Okinawa
Kaikan, Naha

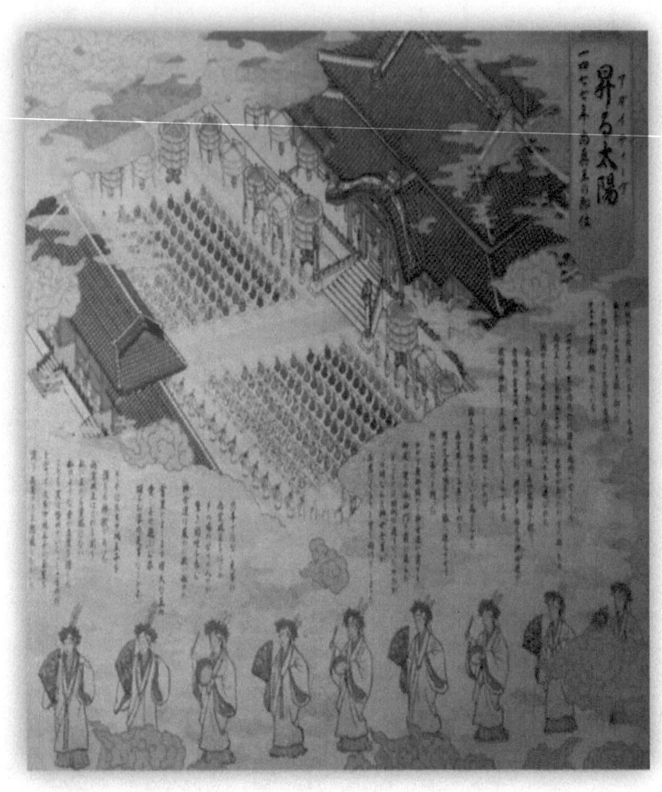

Image of Shuri Castle, Naha

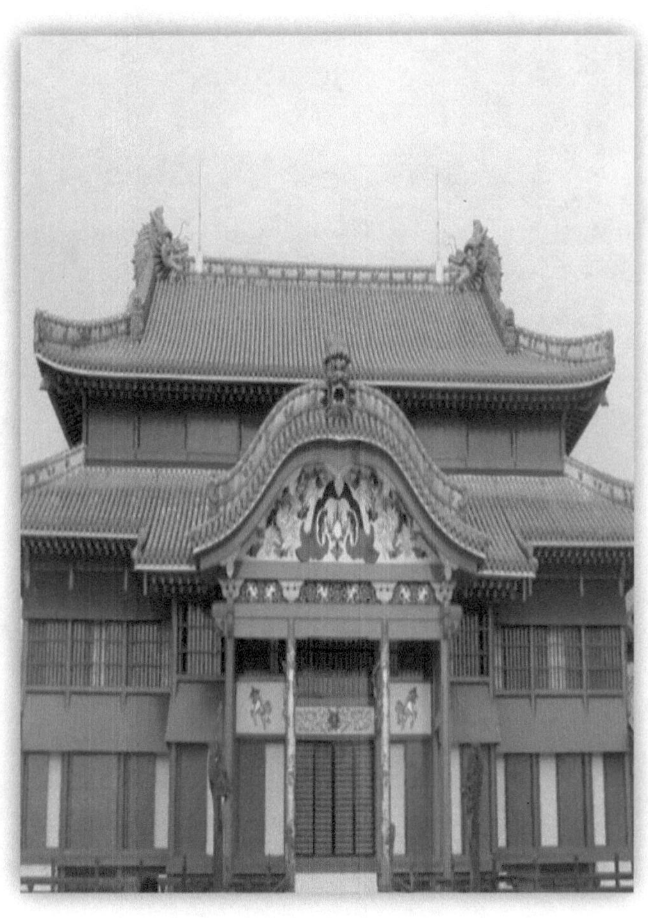

Image of Shuri Castle, Naha

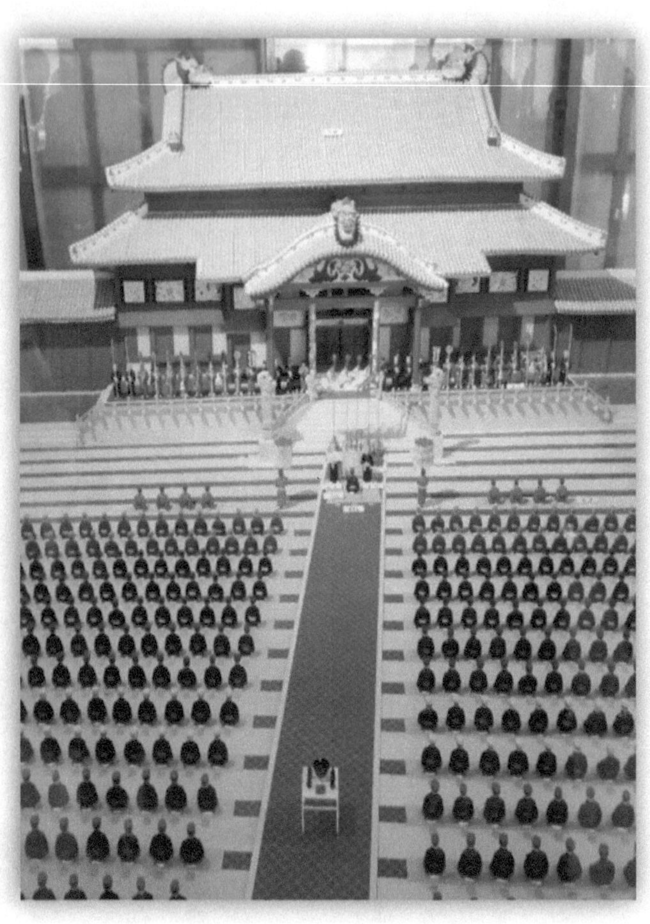

Image of Shuri Castle, Naha

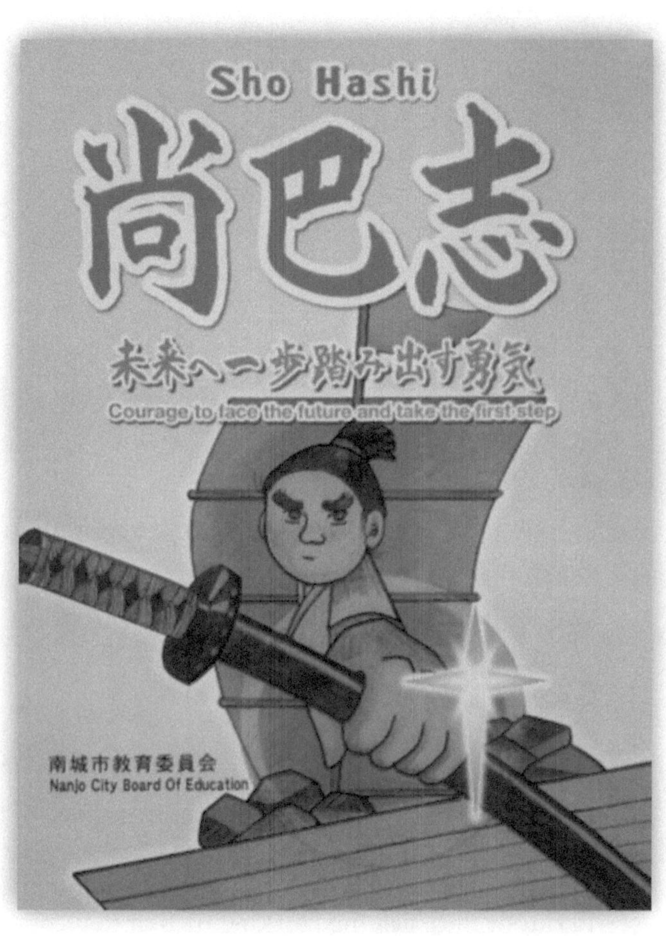

Cover photo of a book on Sho Hashi, first king of the Ryū-kyū kingdom, Sho Hashi was originally from Nanjo, southeast Okinawa

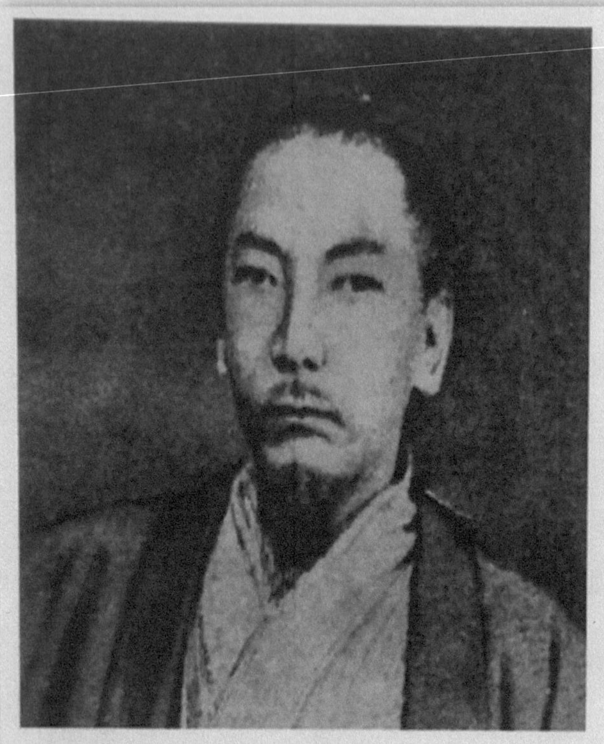

Photo of Sho Tai, the last king of Ryū-kyū,
prefectural history museum, Naha

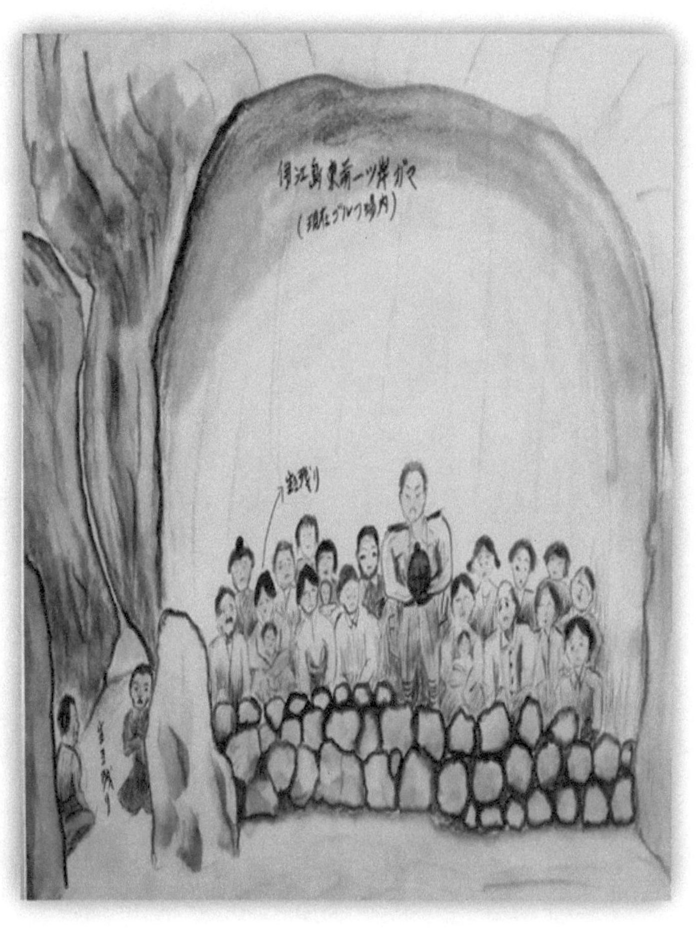

Photo of Okinawans refugees during World War II, Prefectoral Peace Museum, Mabuni Hill, South West Okinawa

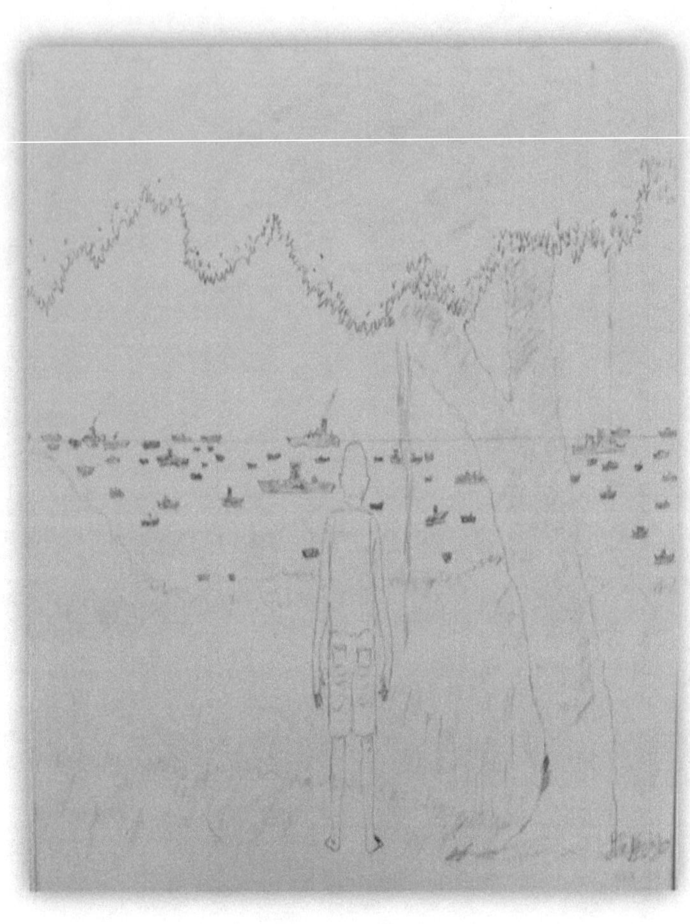

Photo of child watching American ships arriving in
Okinawa during WWII, Prefectoral Peace
Museum, Mabuni Hill, southwest Okinawa

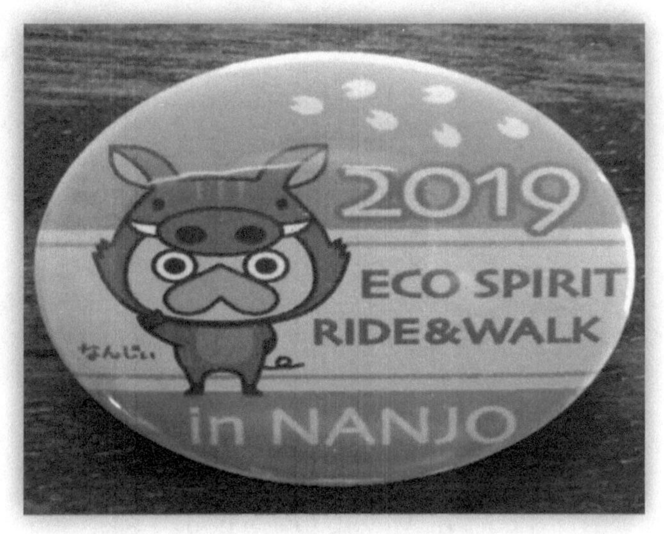

Nanji, mascot of Nanjo, South East Okinawa

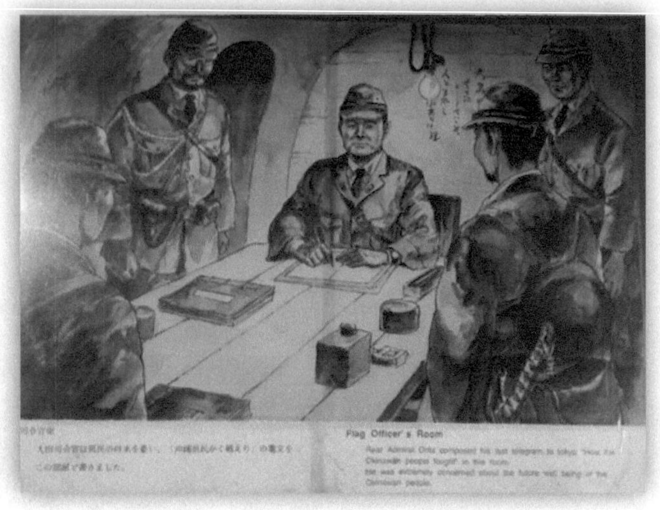

Photo of Minoru Ota, writing a telegraph to recognize the courage of Okinawans in WWII, Underground Navy Museum

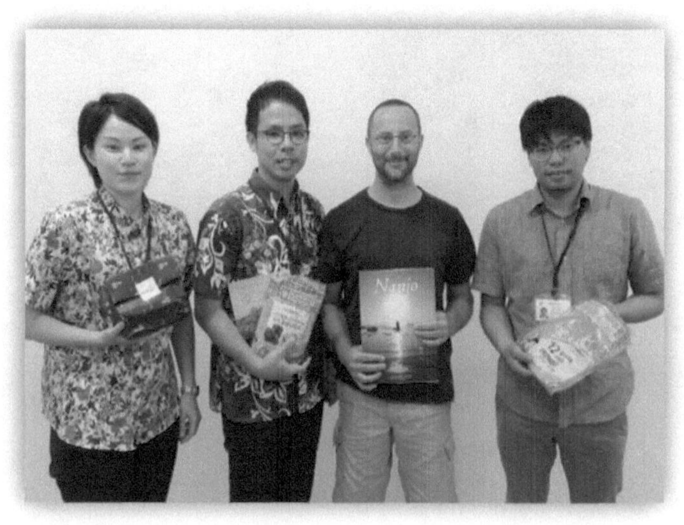

Discussion on Okinawa life, history and culture,
Nanjo City Hall, South East Okinawa

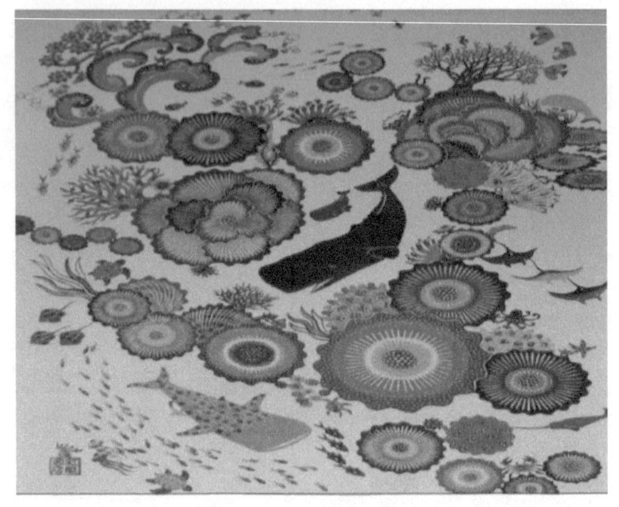

Art Bingata, Okinawa

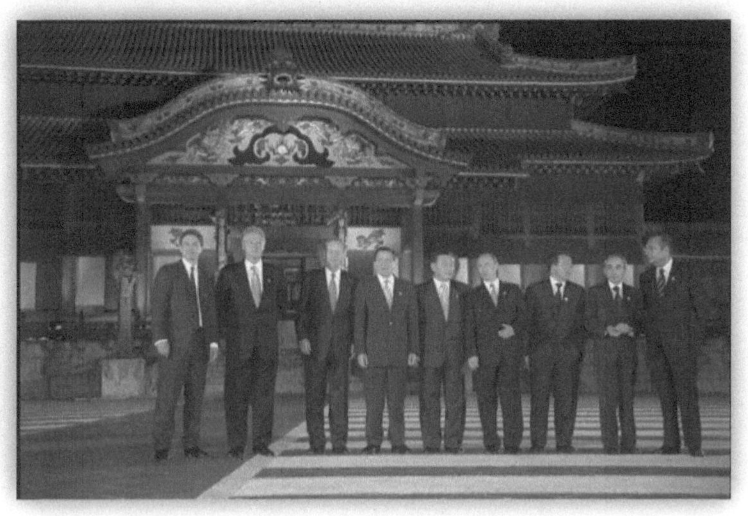

G8 gathered in Okinawa in 2000, in front of Shuri
Castle, Okinawa

In many ways, Okinawa is a unique place in the world.

Honto is the main island of Okinawa and is around 1,200 km2. Naha is the main city. Okinawa has around 160 islands and around 1.4 million inhabitants.

Okinawa is referenced as a World Heritage Site by UNESCO.

Okinawa, nicknamed Japanese Hawaii, it is also a picture postcard landscape: sandy beaches (moreover considered the most beautiful beaches in Japan), an azure blue sea, world-renowned diving spots and places of unique photo shoots.

There are 2,000 species of fish. Manta rays and turtles are also present in the sea.

Tourism has only developed recently. Currently, 6 million tourists visit Okinawa in a year.

The tourists are mainly Japanese, Chinese, Korean and Taiwanese.

Note however that the island is subject to many typhoons, around 45 per year, some of which can be particularly devastating, especially during the period between March and September, a period which is called the "typhoon season".

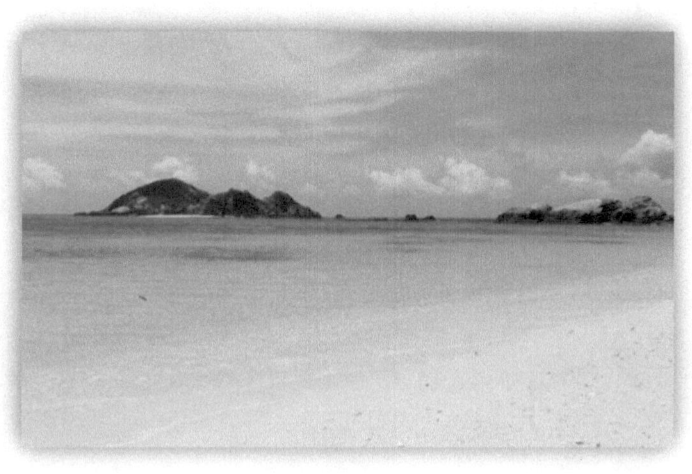

Aharen beach, kerama blue, kerama islands,
tokashiki jima, west of Okinawa, accessible from
the port of Tomari, Naha

In Okinawa, it makes the best longest life in the world: five times less serious disease, with the highest proportion of healthy centenarians.

15% of the planet's super-centenarians (> 110 years old) live in Okinawa while the population of Okinawa represents only 0.002% of the world population.

A sentence is engraved on a rock in Okinawa (see photo on next page), in the village of Ogimi: "At 70 you are just a child, at 80 you are barely a teenager, at 90 if your ancestors call you to join them, ask them to wait until 100 years old, age at which you will reconsider the question ".

There is a much lower proportion of stroke (Cerebral Vascular Accident) and cancer as well as a higher bone density than average.

The centenarians are in good health, in fact only 3% of the centenarians are bedridden.

The longevity of centenarians would not mainly come from genes.

Indeed, Okinawans who moved to Brazil for example have a life expectancy of 17 years lower than those residing in Okinawa.

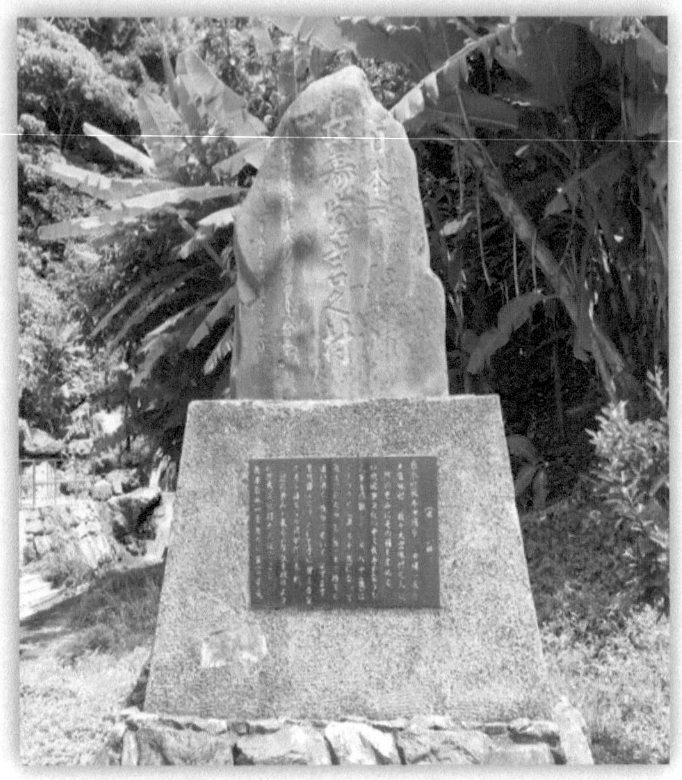

Engraved stone in Ogimi Village, North
Okinawa

"At 70 you are just a child, at 80 you are barely a
teenager, at 90 if your ancestors call you to join
them, ask them to wait until 100 years old, age at
which you will reconsider the question "

But ... there is a but ... because the lifestyles of the older generations are being lost with the younger generations.

After the end of World War II, Okinawa was American until 1972 before being "retroceded" to Japan.

However, 50,000 American soldiers are still in Okinawa, their bases representing around 20% of the surface of the island.

Logistics, planes and helicopters that land and take off with an almost permanent flow adversely affect the carbon footprint of the island.

The soil would be polluted with perfluorooctanesulfonic acid around the American base of the Futenma base in Ginowan.

Other toxic substances were also reportedly discovered around the Kadena base.

American villages have been built and operate according to the American way of life.

However, the Okinawans were not used to this western culture and discovered it almost overnight.

Many young people in Okinawa have now adopted a Western way of life, especially when it comes to fast food.

This generates significant problems of overweight and cardiovascular problems.

Also, part of the younger generations of Okinawa are losing interest in regular sports activities.

Thus, Okinawa is experiencing a decline in life expectancy for the younger generations. People under 50 have the highest per capita hamburger consumption, obesity rate and premature death rate from cardiovascular problems in Japan.

The Okinawan way of life which has been so virtuous is now under threat. It is also said that, henceforth in Okinawa, "the old live old but the young die youg."

However, because of the American influence on the island, baseball is gaining momentum.

Few young people practice karate in Okinawa. Paradoxically, however, it was in Okinawa that karate was born.

Certain inhabitants of the island appreciate this intermingling of cultures and consider that the American influence is a positive contribution, like the contributions of other cultures in Okinawa's past.

Remember that Okinawa, due to its geographical location has already known other influences, such as, for several centuries, from China and then from Japan,

But another part of the population regrets and rejects the American presence and regularly demonstrates for the departure of the GIs.

The elected officials of the Japanese metropolis are not opposed to the American presence at the level of the Japanese prefecture of Okinawa.

The election of Okinawans governors who undertake to fight against the American presence is seen as a setback by the elected officials of the Japanese metropolis, who are then brought "in retaliation", to lower the subsidies of the Japanese state intended for 'Okinawa.

This situation does not facilitate the integration of Okinawa into Japan.

The questionnaire below aims to measure his kotobuki index, that is to say his propensity to live happy over time.

The questionnaire can be completed to have a starting point.

Each question is answered according to the following scale: not at all (1), a little (2), moderately (3), a lot (4) and completely (5).

The questionnaire being composed of 10 questions, the kotobuki index thus varies from 10 in the weakest index to 50 in the highest index.

The questionnaire and the determination of the kotobuki index are simply intended for illustration, without any other pretension.

Two identical questionnaires are presented: the first, on the following page can be carried out upstream of the actions to be decided, and the second, cf. "In summary" below, can be carried out a few months after the implementation of its actions, in order, if necessary, to observe the evolution.

kotobuki index questionnaire	1	2	3	4	5	total
1 / relaxation: do I manage to relax in my daily life?						
2 / the social bond: am I well surrounded in my everyday life?						
3 / work: do I have the feeling that I am helping and that I am useful at work?						
4 / daily diet: do I have good eating habits?						
5 / seniors: are the elders in my environment autonomous and respected?						

kotobuki index questionnaire	1	2	3	4	5	total
6 / interests: do I pursue what passionates me?						
7 / a state of mind: do I regularly take the time to take the time?						
8 / the living environment: is my living environment good?						
9 / the body: do I have regular physical activity?						
10 / nature: do I have the feeling of being in harmony with nature?						
total						

Analysis of the score, according to the kotobuki index:

-        10 to 20: your propensity to live happy over time is potentially moderate as it is. Improvement actions could be carried out.

-        21 to 40: your propensity to live happy over time is present and could however be improved in several aspects.

-        41 to 50: your propensity to live happy over time is strong, but can still be strengthened.

1 / mokuso - relaxation

Okinawans have a strong mental hygiene. They seem appeased. Part of this could be because they take the time to relax and meditate.

Giving yourself a quiet moment in a day is something you probably don't do enough.

Taking care of your mind is probably as important as taking care of your body.

Relaxing, meditating allows you to find coherence, a unity between body and mind.

It comes down to taking the time to listen to yourself, to distance yourself from life events and emotions, to be connected to yourself and to others, living and missing.

Relaxation helps soothe stressful situations. Stress is a obstacle to well-being and undoubtedly an accelerator of aging.

Relaxation makes it possible to manage situations of adversity by relativizing the events that arise.

It also allows you to take the time to contemplate what is around you, "here and now", such as the landscapes, the surrounding noise or the movement of your breathing.

It is also to take the time to realize how lucky one is to have valuable people around you, your family, friends, neighbors.

This makes it possible to perceive things as gifts of life, to be cherished and appreciated.

Karate lessons in Okinawa and around the worl start and end with a short meditation, called "mokuso".

Okinawans cultivate a good emotional balance and seek the well-being of others as much or more than their own well-being.

Life as a couple and family life are based on simplicity, openness and solidarity.

"Ichariba choodee" is a saying in Okinawa which means to treat everyone you meet as if they were family.

Also, "ongaeshi" means to thank by wishing to give back what has been given.

Human relationships are thus healthy and peaceful, embedded with respect, solidarity and common sense.

Helping the other gives a feeling of usefulness and gives meaning to what is done. It is therefore virtuous for the one who gives, as much as it is useful for the one who receives.

An important element is the self-help education that children and adolescents receive in their daily lives by the example of their elders.

The information below comes from several exchanges with Okinawan professionals working on site.

Work is seen as a unique breeding ground for helping each other: it is called "yumaru" in Okinawa.

It consists of rendering services to colleagues, clients, etc. and thus feeling real satisfaction.

Work is thus perceived as a means which makes it possible to render service. Okinawans like to help. So they really like their work.

Remuneration is seen as a consideration, not for oneself, but to help its children, loved ones and family, those around.

Helping each other is giving, but it is also accepting to receive.

Mutual help reinforces the meaning given to what is done, for others and for oneself.

It is also necessary to ensure that there is an adequacy between oneself and the professional activity.

"Pick a job you love and you won't have to work a day in your life." (Confucius)

The risk in case of inadequacy is to consume a lot of energy, to tire excessively and therefore to accelerate its aging.

Likewise, it seems important to keep stress at a reasonable level, so that it is positive and constructive.

To respect everyone is another criteria to feel good at work, whatever the level of responsibility, the beginners as well as the most experienced, the youngest as well as the oldest, to be oneself respected and to respect yourself.

When the work is done, being proud of your work and the tasks performed is a source of satisfaction as well.

You should probably know in advance that everything cannot be perfect in your work environment and that you have to deal with occasionally a little uncomfortable situations.

There is great loyalty to the company in Okinawa, but with regular changes of positions that are privileged within the same company, rather than changing companies.

The time devoted to social activities and festive group outings with colleagues is important and helps to forge and strengthen relationships.

In reality, the notion of the success of the group, of the company, is much more important than the notion of individual success.

"The poor man takes care of his personal interests and the good man takes care of collective interests." (Confucius)

The individual is at the service of the group at the level of the work which is carried out, whatever the level of responsibility and whatever the importance of his work. "The team is the water and the manager is the boat. "(Confucius)

In Okinawa, the weekly working time is 40 hours. The professional subject is taken seriously, with rigor and strong commitment.

The role of work is central for Okinawans, with the wish that this be reconciled with a pleasant daily life, integrating its own organization and family life.

The state of mind observed is positive and constructive, in a mode of identifying solutions rather than in a mode of identifying problems. "Whoever really wants to do something finds a way, others excuses." (Confucius)

Within the company, the teacher-student relationship seems very present. Like learning a martial art, there is a strong relationship between the one who transmits his knowledge and the one who learns, in a harmonious environment marked by respect and fidelity. It brings intimate satisfaction on both sides, pride in transmission and pride in learning.

"Give a man a fish and you feed him for a day, show him how to fish, and you feed him for his whole life." "

In the event of a conflict, 3 ways of reacting exist and seem to be taken from the martial arts: go no sen (react after the aggression), sen no sen (react during the aggression) or sen sen no sen (react even before the aggression).

Knowing how to arbitrate between action and non-action is an action in itself. Choosing the action therefore implies full commitment without hesitation.

Choosing the non action may occasionally be the best possible answer. For example, it may be more appropriate not to outbid in the event of aggression rather than enter into a confrontation.

Non-action is thus an action itself too.

It is accepted, and even encouraged, to procrastinate for a period of time before a decision is made. A first option can come, then another on the opposite direction without this being an issue.

Then, according to the possible options and after several procrastinations a decision is taken and is fully applied.

The approach is circular and not square, like the Japanese flag, and even more the flag of Okinawa prefecture (see photos of the flags below)

Also, the discussions are focused on ondon logic, which we could mean making a "stop in the action", when things do not go as planned, in order to understand and correct the subjects as they go.

This allows the global movement to be in a process of permanent adjustment.

In Asian tradition, it is better to be a reed that bends into the wind rather than an oak that does not bend but ends up being uprooted if the storm is too strong.

"Gujuh taygay" means tough (gujuh) cool (taygay) in the Okinawan language. It is more precisely a mixture of being positive, calm and also objective and rigorous. Deep down, the character is tough and the mindset is cool.

This applies in everyday situations, for example to settle disputes. It will be done in a cool and detached way to a certain extent, and yet with a form of firmness and a genuine willingness to find a solution.

Entrepreneurs who operate in this way generally live in a peaceful way over the long term.

The way in which the Okinawans deal with the subject of the American presence which continues against their will in Okinawa reflects quite well the "gujuh taygay": a pacifist approach in the form but very determined in the substance.

Feeling good about your professional activity is one of the fundamental elements of lasting happiness.

Because of its history and its geographical position, Okinawa is cradled by Chinese influence. Some Chinese or Confucian thoughts have been presented above in this regard.

Japanese flag above

Okinawa Prefecture Flag Above

I would like to clarify that I am neither a nutritionist nor a dietitian. The elements below come from observations of the hygiene of life around dietetics in Okinawa.

Okinawans think "hara hachi bu" before their meal. This means eating only 80% of your perceived fullness, because the stomach takes about 15 minutes to send the signal to the brain that the stomach is full. Thus, when one is already potentially full without knowing it, one would in fact have continued to eat beyond one's satiety threshold.

In other words, at 80% of perception of our satiety, we are no longer hungry, but we do not know it yet, the brain will be informed 15 minutes later.

The people of Okinawa are perhaps one of the only populations around the world to function in this way, deliberately restricting themselves to the amount of food.

This form of frugality makes it possible to keep the figure on the one hand, and on the other hand, to reduce by 20% (100% - 80%) the production of free radicals that are created when we eat.

Free radicals are oxidants, metabolic wastes that oxidize the body like oxidation of a car. The body thus expends energy to deal with and eliminate these free radicals. Free radicals are corrosive wastes that damage the molecules that make us up, which consume energy and therefore accelerate our aging.

The antioxidants which will be mentioned below make it possible to destroy free radicals, and therefore to reduce for example the risk of Macular Degeneration Linked to Age for the eyes or to reduce the oxidation of fats, a process harmful to the body's organization.

In the West, often, in case of stress, a feeling of withdrawal (stopping smoking for example) or annoyance, the reflex to relax can be to fill the stomach by eating, potentially excessively.

However, it is possible to switch from food being source of pleasure, to a food still being source of pleasure but also healthy and useful for the body.

Eating slowly would also have virtues: allowing the brain to realize that the stomach is being full, it also makes it possible to chew more effectively, making the work of the stomach even easier.

Using chopsticks rather than traditional cutlery allows you to eat more slowly.

Nuchi gusui naibitan, which means food ("naibitan") is medicine ("gusui") of life ("nuchi") in the Okinawan language is a formula that considers every food to be a factor of good health.

There is also the expression "kusüi-mun naibitan", which considers food to be medicine for one's body.

It comes down to asking the question: is what I am about to eat good medicine for my body?

Thus, food is seen as a soft and preventive medicine. While in most countries, medicine intervenes a posteriori, in a rather curative manner.

Below are some good practices of Okinawa dietetics, mainly transposable in the West:

• low in sugar (no or little dessert), sugar can be seen as the breeding ground for disease development. Thus, drastically reducing your sugar intake could drastically reduce the risk of disease development.
• low in salt, no addition of salt during cooking and meals
• low in fat (lipids) and calories
• poor in meat, the meat is eaten only once or twice a week, especially with "refute", which means pork, cooked at length and stewed to lighten it as much as possible. Pork is said to contain less cholesterol and fewer calories than chicken or beef
• no or very little dairy
• avoidance of processed foods to limit exposure to chemical and pesticide risks, research into organic and natural products
• oriented vegetables (such as carrots, onions, cabbage, eggplants, peppers) and vegetables
• sweet potato (beni imo), concentrated in slow sugar, and which has the property of filling the stomach. The sweet potato was imported from China by Sokan Noguni, known as the Imo King in Okinawa. This food is still widely used in Okinawan cuisine and is a source of vitamin C, nutrients and beta karotene (anti cancer agent)
• fish rich in omega-3 fatty acid (the human body cannot produce omega 3 on its own), such as eel, tuna and bonito (which looks like tuna), steamed or over low heat , to preserve the maximum of nutrients
• soups, like miso soup

- rice or pasta on the side
- soy through dishes like tofu
- spices such as turmeric, which is said to have many virtues (antioxidant, anti cancer, etc.) and ginger. Spices act as a disinfectant for the body
- chili peppers, such as wasabi yuzu
- thanks to the different ingredients, Okinawan cuisine is known to be "ajikuutaa" which could be translated as "rich in taste"
- matcha green tea, which is said to have the highest proportion of antioxidants in the world, 137 times more antioxidant than conventional green tea
- fruits such as pineapple, mango, orange, star fruit (cut crosswise to keep the star shape), guava (grate), watermelon, papaya

A healthy diet can have the virtue of facilitating the functioning of the intestines.

This allows you to tend towards a satisfactory body mass index, to tend towards your "healthy weight".

Certain foods tend to generate infections in the intestines. On the contrary, vegetables and fruits promote intestinal work and are therefore welcome for the stomach.

This diet could make it possible to partially postpone the programmed obsolescence of the human body.

In Okinawa, food is stored in order that it can not be seen, so that it is not a temptation outside of meals time.

Basically, man comes from frugality, not from opulence. To return to frugality is to return to its origins. It is this moderation that is advocated in Okinawa.

For information, some culinary peculiarities of Okinawa are listed below:

•   goya, which is a bitter cucumber, strong antioxidant, which reduces the level of sugar in the blood, facilitates the regulation of perspiration and provides vitamins, all of which is useful in particular in the summer during high temperatures
•   daikon, which is a large radish
•   mozuku, which are dark brown algae, mozuku contains fucoidan which is known for its strong antioxidant power. Mozuku can be eaten fried (tempura) or with a vinegar sauce
•   nori seaweed
•   umibudo (sea grape)
•   herbs consumed in herbal tea such as mugwort (artemisia)
•   getto leaf (alpinia zerumbet) from the ginger family, which is full of resveratrol, an antioxidant found in grapes
•   nono, fruit with 3 times more vitamin C than oranges. Can be consumed in powder (a brown powder), the nono is prized for its noni juice. The nono would potentially contain substances likely to delay the aging of the skin and protect the body against degenerative diseases such as cancer
•   shikuwasa, a small green citrus fruit rich in citric acid and containing 400 times more polyphenols than other citrus fruits, polyphenol has an antioxidant power
•   roots
•   bagasse, cane sugar powder, known for its virtues that facilitates digestion

- suppon, made from softshell turtle, considered an energy booster

Thus, beyond the content of the plate, it is in fact a global paradigm change in Okinawa when it comes to food.

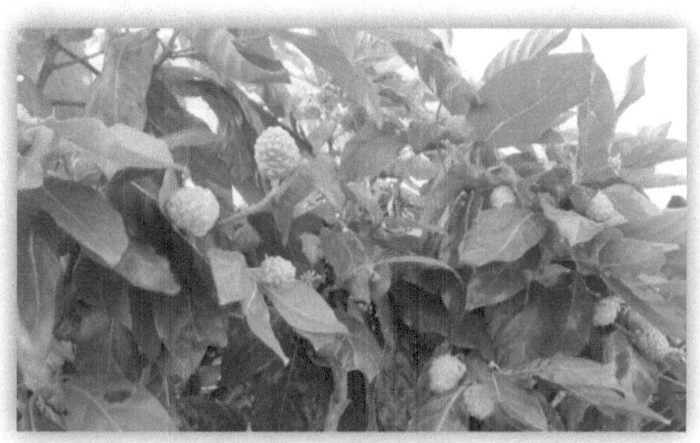

Nono tree, known for its noni juice, Kurkuma
Chinen store, Nanjo, South East Okinawa

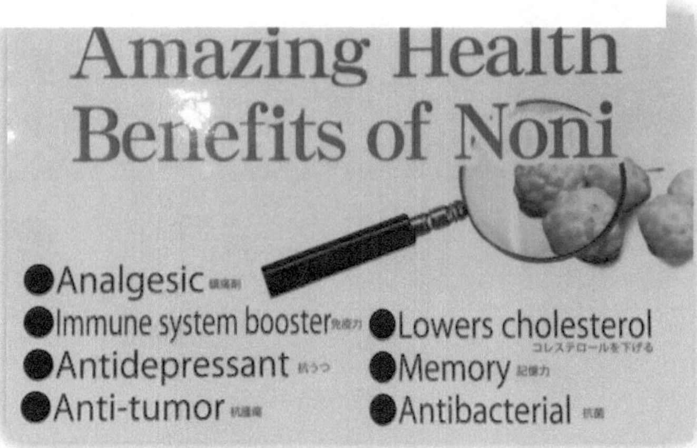

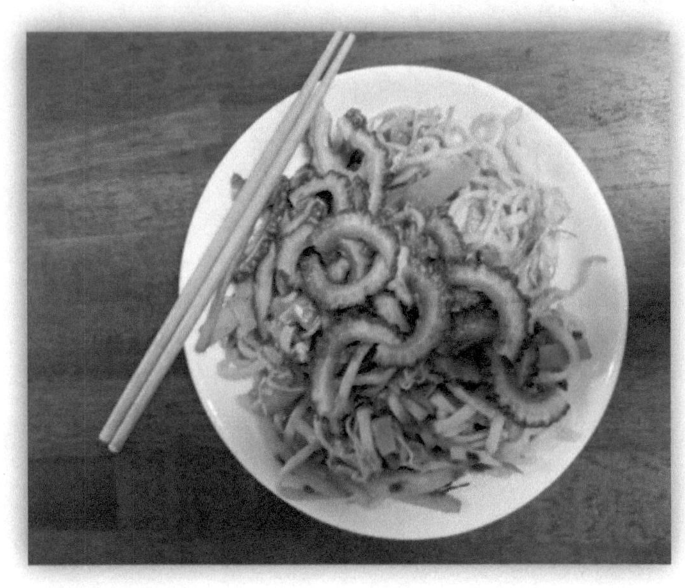

Goya, Okinawan bitter cucumber

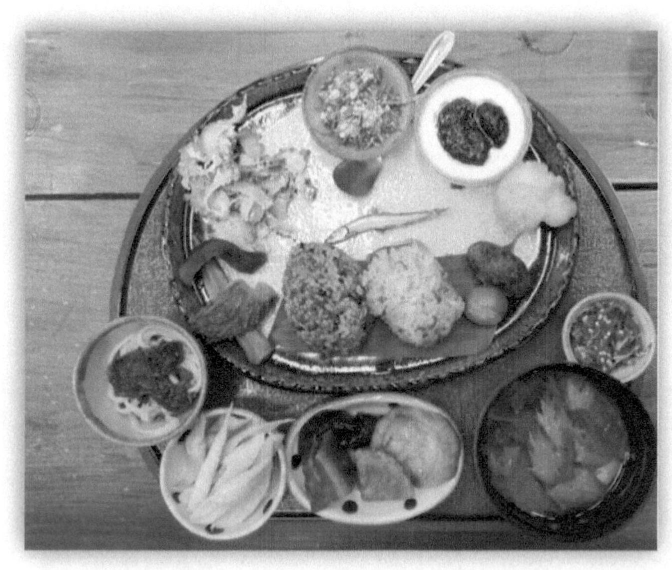

Restaurant, Emi no mise, longevity lunch, centenarians' meal, Ogimi Village, North Okinawa

Seniors are seen in Okinawa as "ayakaru", which means "lucky charm".

Elders often live with their children and family, either in the same house, with a dedicated floor, or in a house nearby.

In this way, there is no isolation of seniors and the intergenerational links are very strong.

Living well in your home seems almost sacred. Two Shīsā, "siisaa" in the Okinawan language, representing an animal half lion and half dog, protect each house.

We will find there, outside in front of the main door or on the roof, on the right, the male shīsā with his mouth open to scare evil spirits, and on the left, the female shīsā with his mouth closed to keep the good ones in the house.

The youngest help the seniors by allowing them to live close to them and the seniors help the younger ones.

Seniors participate in family life with multiple services such as babysitting, preparing meals or taking care of the laundry and the cleanliness of the house. This is an intergenerational mutual help.

Everyone is fundamentally a winner: the children and grandchildren are grateful for this helping hand from their elders, and the seniors are also winners because it gives them activity and usefulness, all in a spirit of family mutual support.

In reality, it is in fact about loving and being loved within the family, a feeling that allows you to feel good, to feel wanted, useful, expected and thus to give meaning to your life.

In fact, there are very few retirement homes in Okinawa.

They are seniors who love life: "ping ping colori" as one old man from the island says with a smile.

Elders also remain involved in professional activities or as a volunteer. It is for this reason that the word "retirement" has no real translation in the Okinawan language.

Thus, active life continues throughout life. This could be selling beach items in stores, selling vegetables to restaurants or other activities.

Elderly people work an estimated 1/4 time job, as a contribution to society, leads to respect for assets and therefore allows seniors to be more integrated into society.

The "moai" is very of the Okinawans everyday life. It is a network of geographically close friends, with regular meetings. The moai plays an important role in the socialization of elders. The discussions can relate to family life or to the studies of the grandchildren. It can also relate to financial assistance.

This notion of group allows everyone to be able to count on a strong network, where everyone can help and be helped.

Elders continue to exercise even in old age. It is also not uncommon to see centenarians continue to practice karate in groups, less physically than the youngest practitioners, but in a more fluid and internal way.

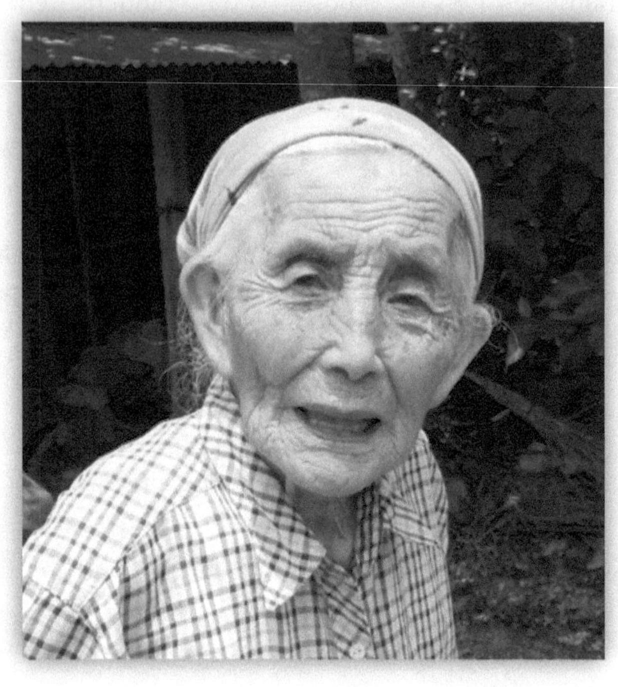

Centennial taking care of its garden, Ogimi
Village, North Okinawa

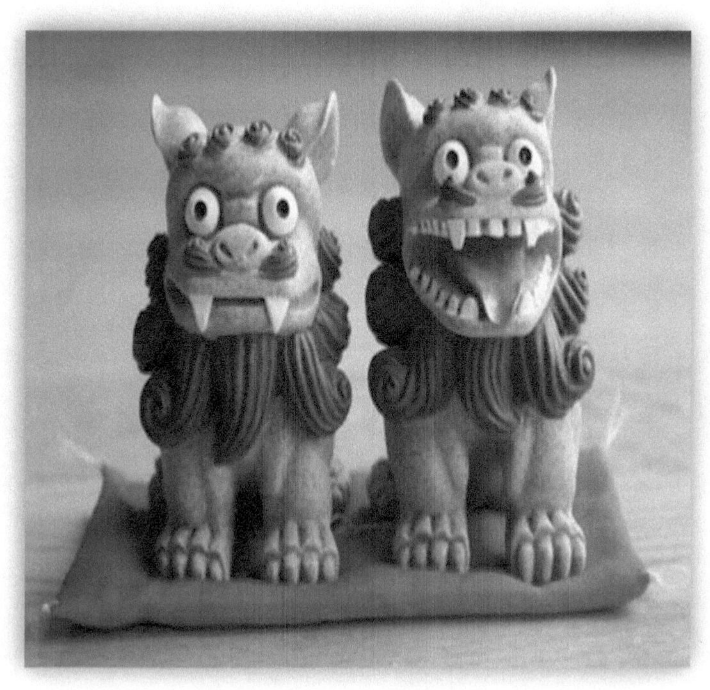

Shīsā, Okinawa

It is about passion, reason for being, vocation, about the reason why we get up in the morning.

Finding your "ikigai" comes down to being attentive to what you love, to discover it, before and in order to be able to achieve it.

"Ikigaï" does not really have a translation, and is at the crossroads between his passions, his life mission, his vocation and even his profession.

This is a concept known throughout Japan.

This can concern its job (and especially the meaning one gives to its job), family, friends, sports, cultural or artistic hobbies, volunteering, religious activities, reading etc.

After having identified it, it is a question of organizing oneself to live it, which makes it possible to fully realize oneself to be happy because connected to what is deep down.

Note that his "ikigai" can evolve over time and over his life course.

"uchina taimu" could be translated into the Okinawan language by taking the time to take the time.

We also hear "nankurunaisa" which means "take things as they come". It is a positive philosophy of life. It is also caring for the spiritual as much or more than the material.

Material accumulation does not seem to be a priority in Okinawa. It is rather a matter of living simply, almost in a minimalist version when it comes to the material organization.

Moreover, the inhabitants of Okinawa do not seem attached to a specific goal. As Hesna Cailliau indicates in her book "The Goldfish Paradox", "The fixation on a goal presents two major drawbacks: it is a source of tension which squanders the vital energy of man and consequently shortens his life, it does not allow us to see what is happening at ground level and therefore to seize the opportunities that arise. "

Okinawans have a basic principle: land, people and life could not have existed. Thus, the very fact of existing is taken positively.

It comes down to cultivating the joy of living and one's sense of humor, of smiling (vitamin S / Smile), of laughing, singing, dancing, playing or listening to music. The people of Okinawa are very fond of festivals and organize them throughout the year. The festivals are following the rhythm of the solar calendar and the seasons of crops. For example, the Memorial Day of the Missing, called Obon, which is held in August, could potentially take place on a different date between Okinawa and the Japanese metropolis.

It's about enjoying the present moment, with ease, taking advantage of what is, not what could have been, taking the time to take the time, not to do several things at the same time.

Okinawans try not to waste energy in nervousness, resentment and animosity.

Negative emotions are seen as temporary emotions, like clouds that pass through the sky and disappear.

Thus, energy is not consumed to deal with negative emotions, which would presumably accelerate aging.

For example, if a noise is unpleasant outside, this noise will not necessarily be perceived as annoying and unpleasant noise, but only as noise, which it is, no more.

This mode of operation makes it possible not to cling to annoying things, but to simply note their existence and let them slide.

Likewise, it comes down to being in a logic of permanent personal improvement, to be aligned between the person you are, your lifestyle and your values, to adapt naturally to new situations, without clinging to habits for fear of change.

It also allows for strong resilience in the face of adversity.

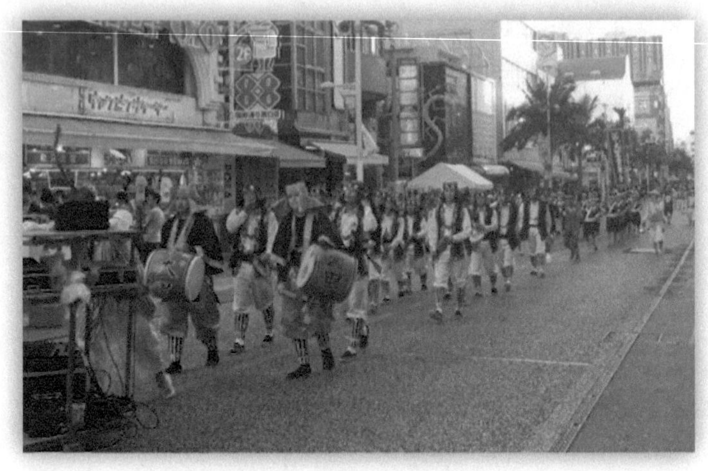

Above and below, Festival Eisa, kokusai dori,
Naha

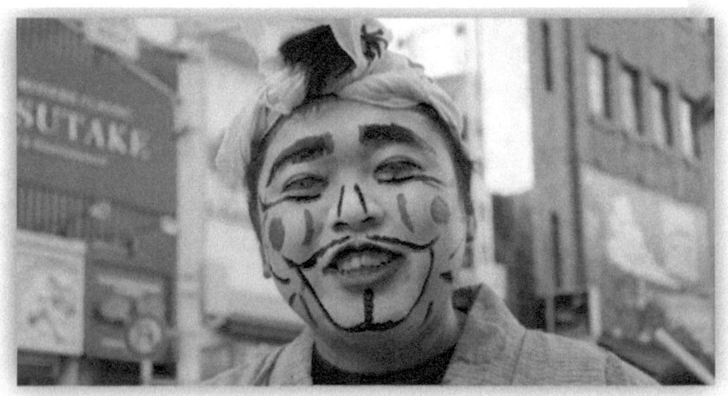

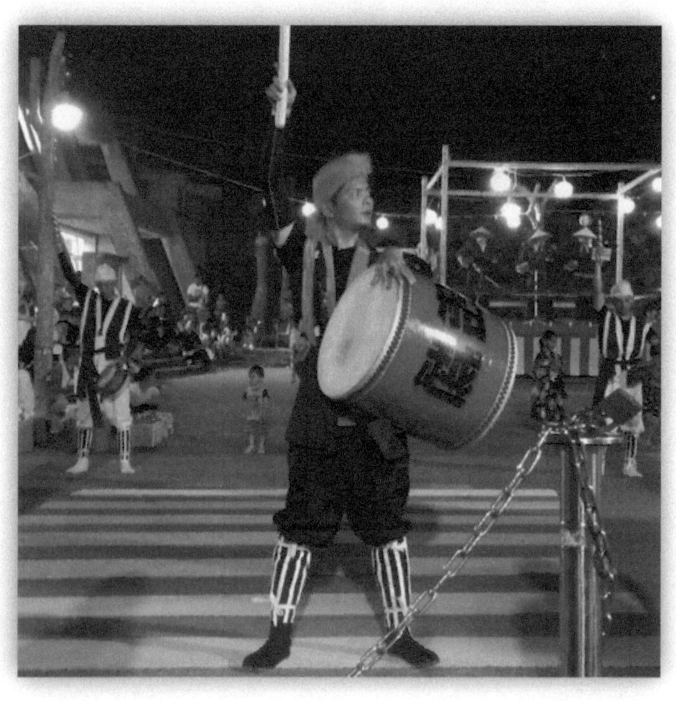

Eisa Festival, in front of the Nanjo, Funakoshi
Community Center, Tamagusuku, Nanjo, South
East Okinawa

"Churasan" means "beautiful place" in the Okinawan language.

Brightness is conducive to the production of vitamin D, which itself is important for protecting the body.

Our body would need 10 to 15 minutes of sun exposure twice a week.

However, you should protect your skin to avoid sunburn, which is harmful to the skin. Indeed, the organism sets out to replace dead skin cells with new ones, which requires energy from the body, and therefore mechanically accelerates its aging, beyond the risk of subsequent development of a skin disease.

Generally stable temperatures can also play a role, when the temperature does not vary by a very large amplitude between seasons.

Living in an environment with reduced pollution is a major factor in health and well-being. The World Health Organization indicates that there are more premature deaths linked to pollution than linked to tobacco.

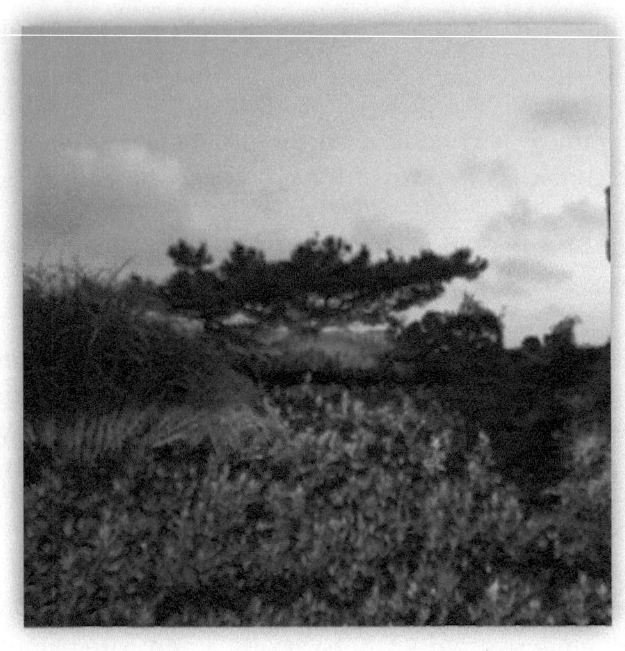

In front of our rental house, Tamagusuku,
Nanjo, South East Okinawa

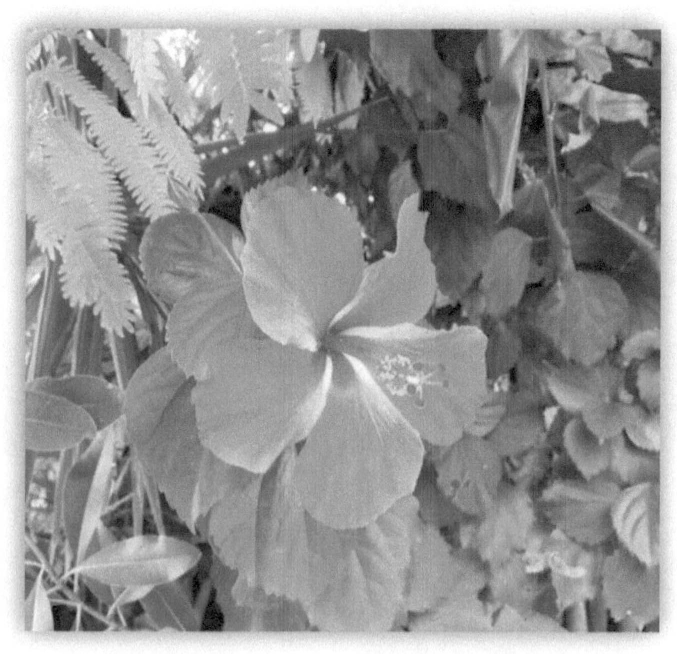

Hibiscus flower, Okinawa

Taking care of your body and health is an integral part of the Okinawan way of life.

Okinawans are on standby in relation to the signals (pain, blockages, etc.) that the body sends.

They consider that our body is made up of 35,000 trillion cells. They thank their cells and the different parts of the body, considering that it is thanks to their body that we can live and practice our activities.

It is about taking care of your body and preventing it from risks (like tobacco, etc.).

The daily physical practice is part of the habits of the inhabitants of Okinawa, integrating a solicitation of the heart by the increase of the heart rate.

It is considered that our body should be able to live approximately and on average up to 90 years. However, on average, the actual life expectancy observed is rather around 75 to 80 years. Thus, it would be possible to gain 10 to 15 more years of a satisfying life by living the first 75 to 80 years a little differently.

This requires daily exercise, for example climbing stairs rather than taking the elevator, walking rather than taking the car.

The credo of karate, whose birthplace is in Okinawa, is "a healthy mind in a healthy body".

Here are some beneficial effects of karate, which are similar for other martial arts and many other physical activities:

- allows you to be connected to your body
- cardiovascular exercises that help maintain good health
- helps balance and posture
- staying calm under pressure, which allows you to be less tense in the face of difficulties in everyday life
- improves self-confidence
- discipline that can be practiced as a family
- allows you to forge new friendships
- healthy lifestyle
- regardless of gender, religion or social level

Physical fatigue is also helpful for quality sleep.

Here are some peculiarities of karate in Okinawa that I was able to identify on site:

• karate in Okinawa goes far beyond sport, even goes beyond martial art, it's a real art of living
• the dojo is often located at the sensei's home
• a contribution to the costs is given to the senseiu for his instruction
• the protocol is very important (for example the greeting at the entrance of the dojo when arriving and leaving, as well as the standing and seated greeting) and the presence of a "lineage table" at the dojo, which is a form of family tree previous sensei which may, depending on the style of karate practiced, date back to the 1700s
• small group of students but very close, almost a family, with the sensei. A moment during the course is also dedicated to personal time between the sensei and each student. The bond is very strong between the students too
• personal warm-up before the start of the course and the importance of muscle work (makiwara, chiichi, sachii, sandbag, etc.) and the importance of strengthening, especially forearms
• regular practice of kobudō (bo, saï and others) very related to karate
• a lot of repetitions of movements to find anchorage and automatism
• practitioners in Okinawa don't say "oss" like in the Japanese metropolis and around the world to nod and show commitment to self-improvement, but rather say "hai"

• Gichin Funakoshi is not very celebrated in Okinawa. The shotokan style, of which he is the founder, is very present in the Japanese metropolis and around the world, but is not very present on the island. Gichin Funakoshi, who is originally from Okinawa, can be perceived as the investigator of the japonization of Okinawan karate, a step which he undoubtedly considered necessary to allow a democratization of karate beyond Okinawa

• less interest in karate on the part of the younger generations (more interested in other activities such as, for example, baseball) and therefore a medium-term challenge to perpetuate karate on site in Okinawa

• "It is the state of mind, more than the technique, which constitutes the essence and the peculiarity of Okinawan karate"

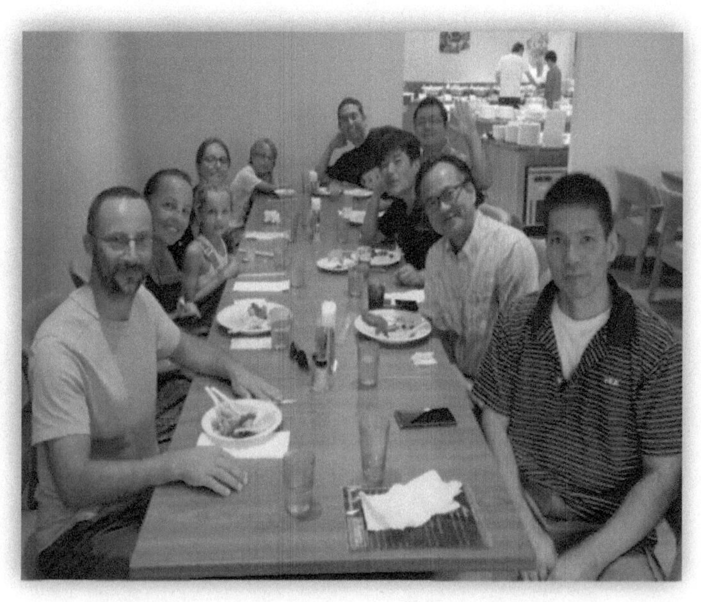

Pacific Hotel, Naha, with Takuya Kawasaki and
members of the Okinawa Karatedō Kobudō
Shōrin-ryū Bushinkan dojo

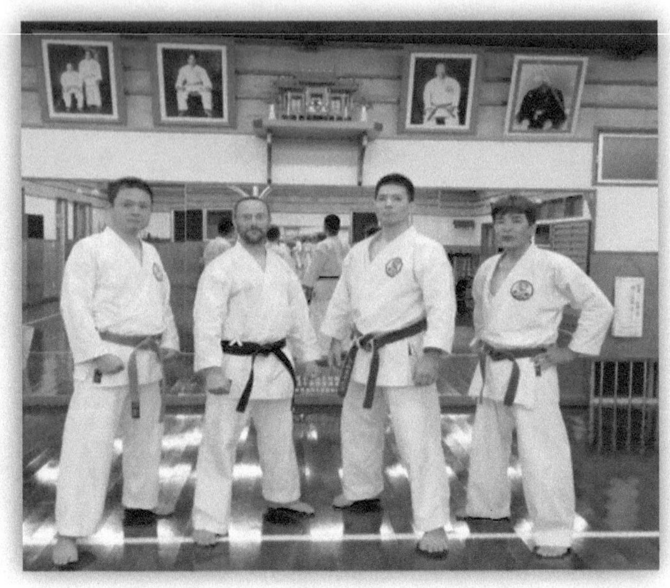

Dojo - with Takuya Kawasaki and members of
the Okinawa Karatedō Kobudō Shōrin-ryū
Bushinkan dojo, Nanjo-city, southeast Okinawa

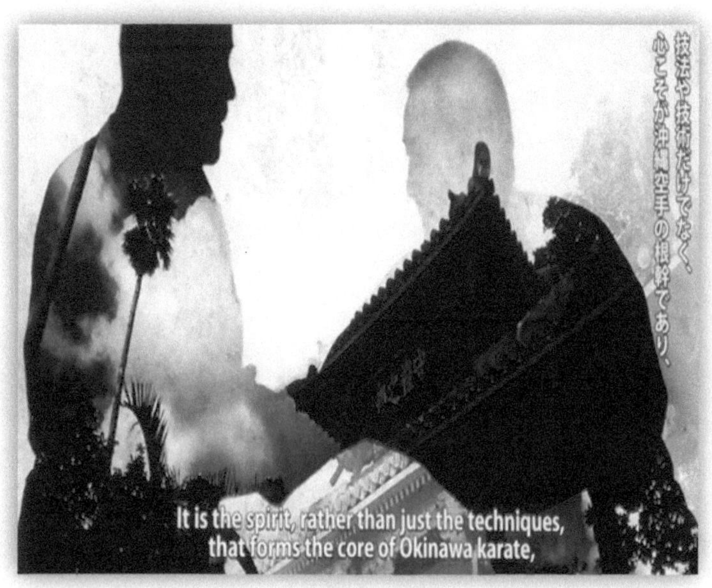

Kaikan - OKIC (Okinawa Karate Information Center), Naha

Regarding spiritual beliefs, there is a belief in Okinawa that differs from Shintoism and Buddhism, which are predominant in the Japanese metropolis. This belief is based on nature itself, with places of contemplation called utaki.

Man is seen in Okinawa as part of the universe, not as the center of the universe. Man is therefore part of a great whole.

It takes humility to recognize that one is part of a larger whole than oneslef, and that you are not the center of that whole, and that this whole outweight the individual.

Thus, less weight is put on the individual shoulders when things do not go quite as desired.

The human body is made up of 90% water, water is nature, therefore our body is nature.

Okinawans consider nature to be a sacred good. Islands, like Kudaka, are moreover entirely considered sacred natural places.

Decisions of everyday life in Okinawa take into account the subject of nature and the environment in a natural way. Many Okinawa residents grow vegetables in their own gardens, which strengthens their connection with nature.

The tombs, in the shape of a turtle, are very large, allowing families to gather together, and are not grouped together in a cemetery, but positioned individually in nature.

His own death and the deaths of relatives do not seem to be a source of anxiety in Okinawa.

Life is seen as coming from nature, death is seen as returning to nature, allowing rebirth from nature again.

This continuity in life favors Okinawans not to focus on the cosmetic appearance of their body, considering that it only accompanies them for a given time. This thus reduces the perception of small physical defaults or imperfections.

It also minimizes the power consumption from its body that might otherwise exist.

Because of this continuity, it is rare to hear in Okinawa "we only have one life" or to see people wanting at all costs to make their mark (political, major project, business, etc) on earth.

So things are done, but in a peaceful and peaceful way, without having the feeling of running after time.

This is undoubtedly one of the keys to happiness that is felt in a very palpable way in Okinawa.

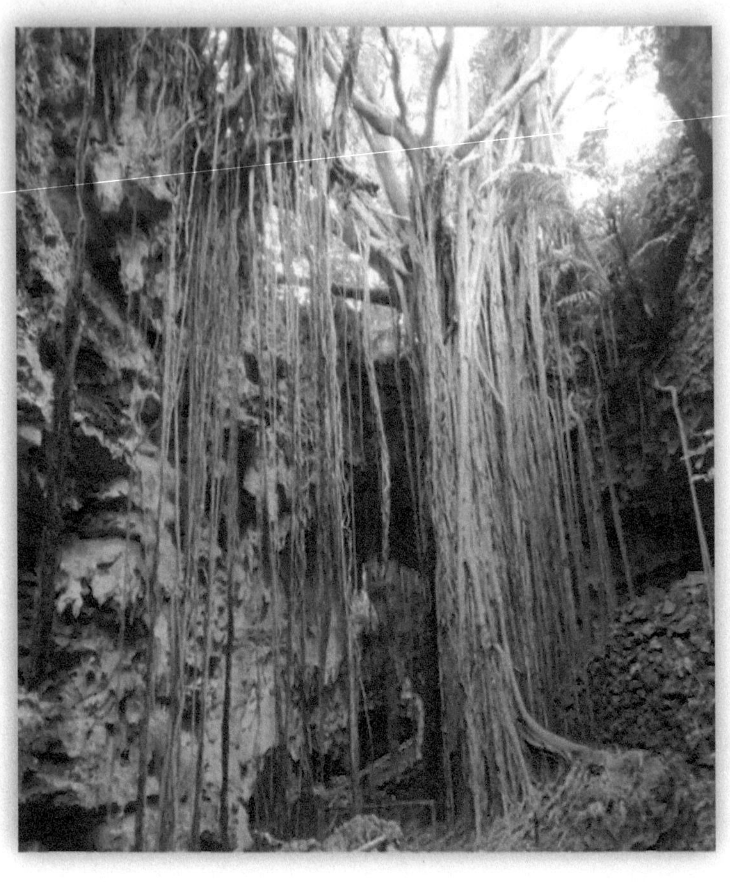

Valley of Gangala, Nanjo, South East Okinawa

"The walking trees"

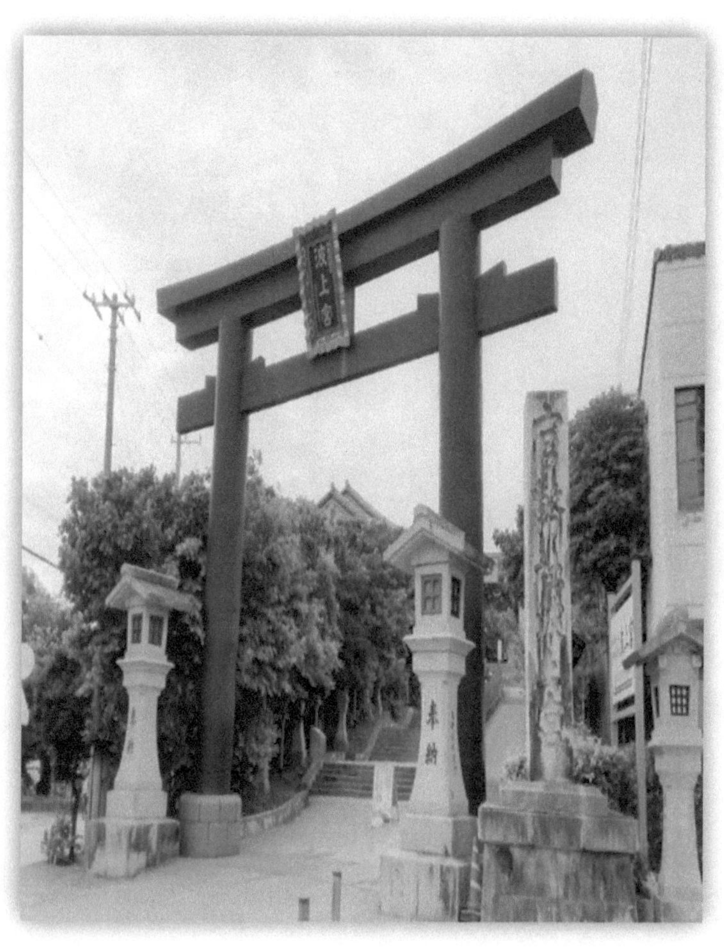

Naminoue temple, Naha

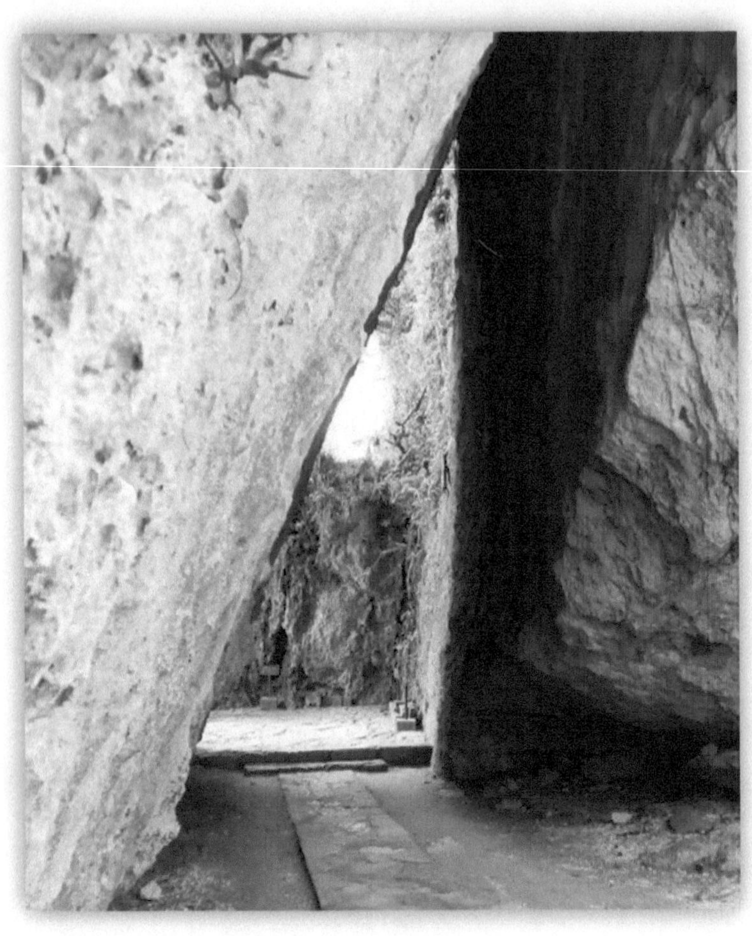

Sefa utaki, sacred site of the kingdom Ryū-kyū,South
East Okinawa

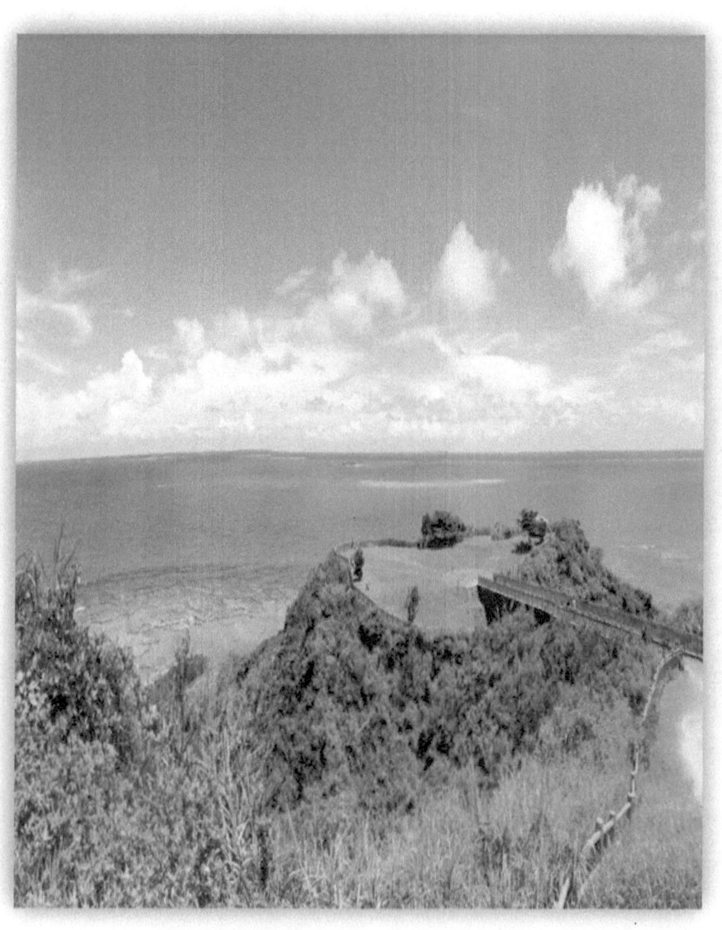

Cap Chinen, South East Okinawa

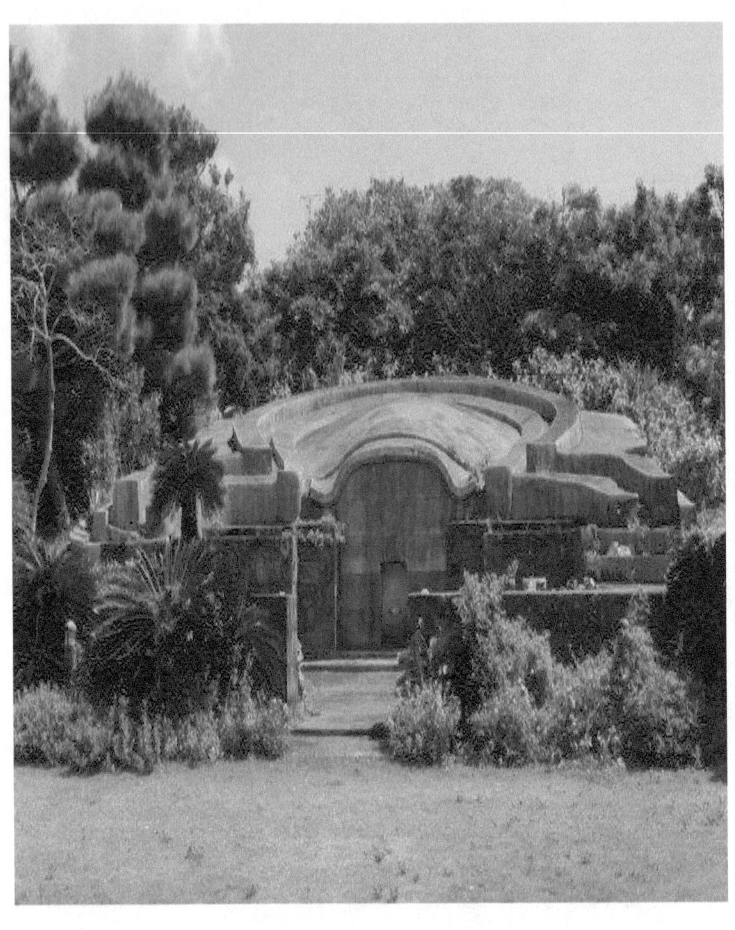

Kameko baka, tumbs, from Okinawa, falls in the
shape of a turtle shell

the the 10 keys of Okinawa:

1 / mokuso - relaxation

2 / ichariba choodee - social link

3 / yumaru - to help at work to feel useful

4 / nuchui gusui naibitan - a dietetic medicine of life

5 / ayakaru - respect for seniors

6 / ikigaï - find and pursue your passion

7 / uchina taimu - a state of mind

8 / churasan - a good living environment

9 / ganjyuu - maintenance of his body

10 / kudaka - the connection with nature

The the 10 keys of Okinawa are translated below into examples of personal decisions in its everyday life, considering that everyone is at the helm of their art of living.

1 / relax

2 / treat everyone as if they were family

3 / helping at work to feel useful

4 / eat at 80% of your satiety

5 / respect seniors

6 / live your passions

7 / follow a positive life philosophy

8 / live in a good environment

9 / maintain your body

10 / be in touch with nature

NB: do not hesitate to fill again the kotobuki index questionnaire (see below) a few months after having implemented the decisions relating to your art of living.

kotobuki index questionnaire	1	2	3	4	5	total
1 / relaxation: do I manage to relax in my daily life?						
2 / the social bond: am I well surrounded in my everyday life?						
3 / work: do I have the feeling that I am helping and that I am useful at work?						
4 / daily diet: do I have good eating habits?						
5 / seniors: are the elders in my environment autonomous and respected?						

kotobuki index questionnaire	1	2	3	4	5	total
6 / interests: do I pursue what passionates me?						
7 / a state of mind: do I regularly take the time to take the time?						
8 / the living environment: is my living environment good?						
9 / the body: do I have regular physical activity?						
10 / nature: do I have the feeling of being in harmony with nature?						
total						

Analysis of the score, according to the kotobuki index:

-	10 to 20: your propensity to live happy over time is potentially moderate as it is. Improvement actions could be carried out.

-	21 to 40: your propensity to live happy over time is present and could however be improved in several aspects.

-	41 to 50: your propensity to live happy over time is strong, but can still be strengthened.

Okinawa is a unique island, which has virtuous practices, with a well-being that is felt and a unique philosophy of life.

But the younger generations don't necessarily follow the way of life of their elders less.

Thus, the vocation of this book is to ensure that these keys, these secrets, which continue to be put into practice, in particular by the most senior part of the population, are not lost and that, on the contrary, this art of living can continue into the future, in Okinawa and beyond Okinawa.

"kotobuki", the title of the book, means "long life" in the Okinawan language

"kotobuki", the title of the book, means "long life" in the Okinawan language

bibliography

Buettner Dan, Blue Zones, 9 lessons for living longer

Cailliau Hesna, The Goldfish Paradox

Curtay Jean-Paul, Okinawa, a global program for better living

Dalai Lama, The Art of Happiness

David-Néel Alexandra, Journey of a Parisian to Lhassa

Dufour Anne, Okinawa, the best diet in the world

Greger Michael, How not to die

Johnston Jeremiah, Okinawa Island Tour

Juster Jean-Charles, Past and present of the Okinawan performing arts

Marx Thierry, The Strategy of the Dragonfly

Puech Michel and Wang Hélène, The Philosophy of the Tatami

Suzuki Makato, Willcox Craig, Willcox Bradley, the Okinawa way

Williamson Mark, Action for Happiness

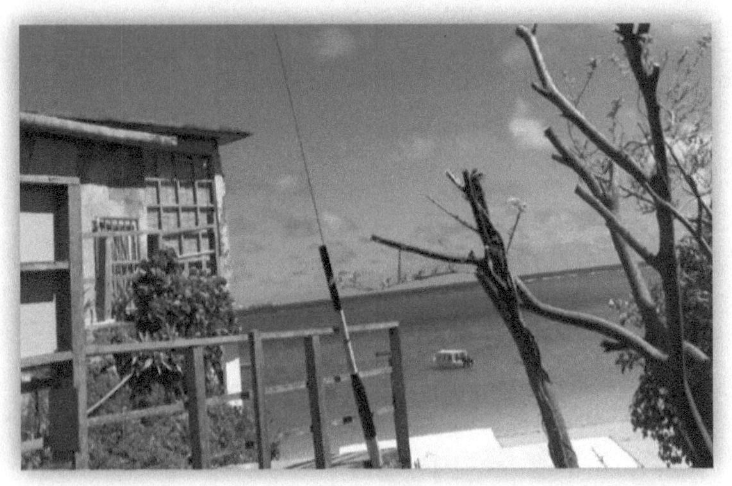

Mibaru beach, Tamagusuku, Nanjo, South East
Okinawa

front cover: photo when we arrived in Okinawa, Mibaru beach, Tamagusuku, Nanjo, South East Okinawa

Table of Contents

contact

contact@okinawa-kotobuki.com

International Standard Book Number (ISBN)

ISBN: 978-2-9572022-2-5

EAN: 9782957202225

OVHcloud

reference: PP_FR9490936 and FR34538072

domain: okinawa-kotobuki.com

E-mail :contact@okinawa-kotobuki.com

Secure and AFNOR certified archiving (NF Z 42-013 standard NF 461 mark)

INPI reference: DSO2020005391

INPI, National Institute of Intellectual Property

"The Intellectual Property Code prohibits copies or reproductions intended for collective use. Any full or partial representation or reproduction made by any means whatsoever, without the consent of the author or his successors in title, is illegal and constitutes an infringement"

Administered by WIPO, the World Intellectual Property Organization, the Berne Convention establishes the fundamental principles that signatory states must guarantee in their copyright policies and laws. Copyright protection is granted to works in the178 countries parties to this Convention.

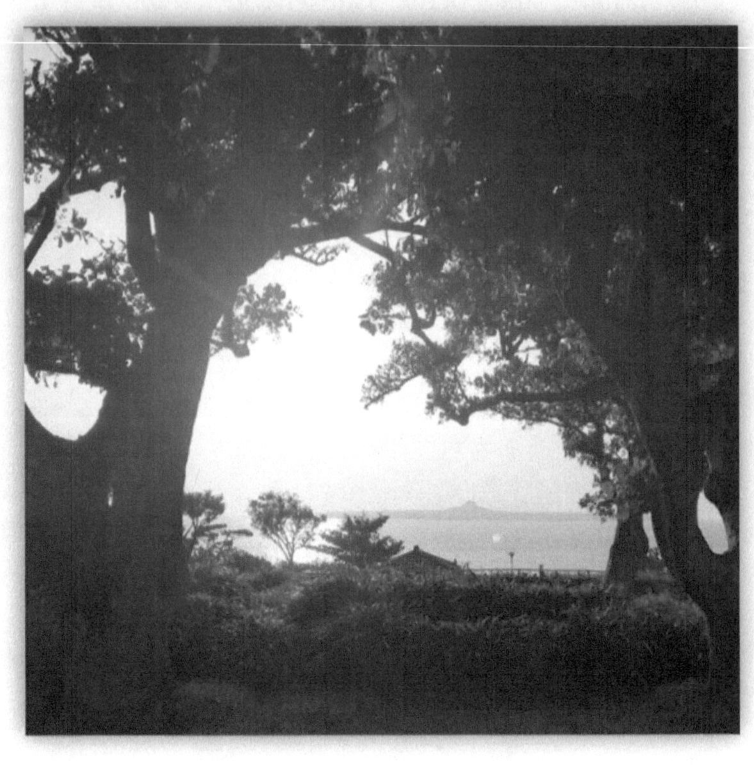

Churaumi Aquarium Park, Motobu, Northwest
Okinawa

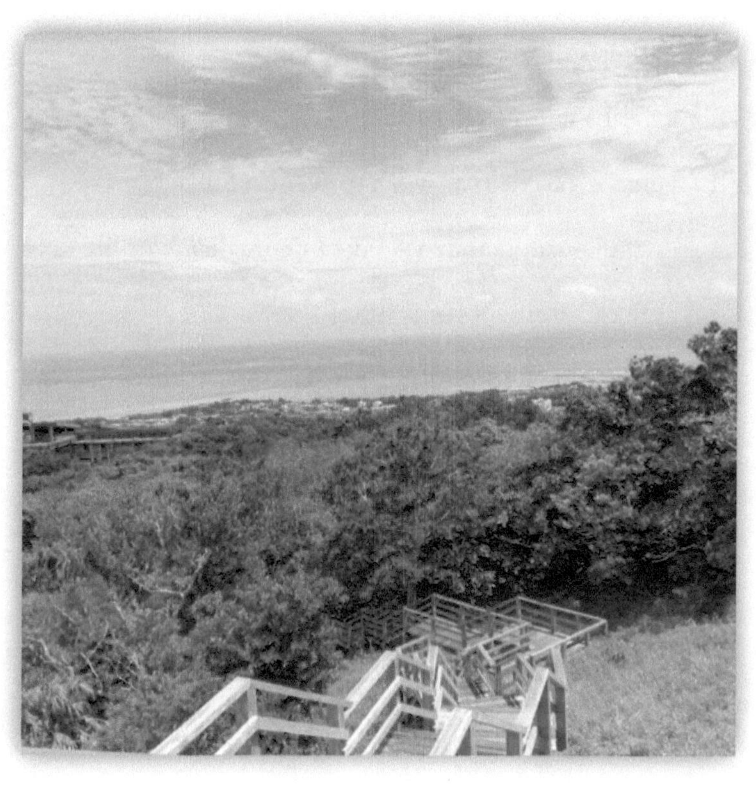

View from Tamagusuku Gusuku Castle, Nanjo, South East Okinawa

to remember

the 10 keys of Okinawa to live happy

1 / mokuso - relaxation

2 / ichariba choodee - social link

3 / yumaru - to help at work to feel useful

4 / nuchui gusui naibitan - a dietetic medicine of life

5 / ayakaru - respect for seniors

6 / ikigaï - find and pursue your passion

7 / uchina taimu - a state of mind

8 / churasan - a good living environment

9 / ganjyuu - maintenance of his body

10 / kudaka - the connection with nature

9 782957 202225